Sugar Addiction

A Guide to the Causes & Consequences
of Sugar Addiction and How to Cure It

J. A. Sutton

J. A. Sutton Copyright © 2015

Disclaimer

No part of this publication may be reproduced or transmitted in any form or by any means, mechanical or electronic, including photocopying or recording, or by any information storage and retrieval system, or transmitted by email without permission in writing from the publisher.

While all attempts and efforts have been made to verify the information held within this publication, neither the author nor the publisher assumes any responsibility for errors, omissions, or opposing interpretations of the content herein.

This book is for entertainment purposes only. The views expressed are those of the author alone, and should not be taken as expert instruction or commands. The reader of this book is responsible for his or her own actions when it comes to reading the book.

Adherence to all applicable laws and regulations, including international, federal, state, and local governing professional licensing, business practices, advertising, and all other aspects of doing business in the US, Canada, or any other jurisdiction is the sole responsibility of the purchaser or reader.

Neither the author nor the publisher assumes any responsibility or liability whatsoever on the behalf of the purchaser or reader of these materials.

Any received slight of any individual or organization is purely unintentional.

Contents

Introduction

First and foremost I want to thank you for purchasing the book, "SUGAR ADDICTION – A Guide to the Causes & Consequences of Sugar Addiction and How to Cure It".

In this book you will learn how to recognize the symptoms of sugar addiction and identify if you or a family member has a problem with sugar. Not everyone who reads this book will be addicted to sugar, but it is likely that the majority will be consuming far more sugar than is healthy for them on a daily basis.

Many people suffer with an addiction to sugar and it is far more common than most of us realize. Whilst reading through these pages you may identify many symptoms of excess sugar consumption within yourself and those close to you which will, I hope, give you the opportunity to address these issues and make changes to your diet so you can alleviate any of the health problems which you may be experiencing.

Thanks again for purchasing this book! I hope you enjoy it, and please leave a review once you are finished.

Chapter 1 – What is a Sugar Addiction?

Contrary to what many people believe, a sugar addiction is not restricted to people who consume large quantities of sweets, cakes and other sugar filled treats. Due to the high levels of sugars hidden within the convenience foods which currently fill the supermarket shelves, a sugar addition is extremely common yet worryingly, it is often undiagnosed.

Even the so called healthy foods such as yoghurts, dietary foods, fresh fruit juices and smoothies and those labelled as low fat, often contain more sugar than is good for us, but this is mostly hidden under the guise of different names.

Only a small percentage of the population will recognize that they could have a problem with sugar addiction while the rest of us are either blissfully unaware or in a constant state of denial.

Sugar affects us physically, emotionally and neurologically, and while it can be easy to recognize the physical symptoms once they are pointed out, the idea that we can have an emotional and also neurological based addiction is only rarely considered.

This three pronged attack makes it a difficult addiction to cure, especially when so many food manufacturers do such a good job of hiding it behind scientific names or, even worst, a combination of letters and numbers which give no indication as to what they really are, but it is possible to learn to control your sugar intake.

So how and why do we become addicted in the first place?

Most people can identify with the experience of feeling upset or sad and reaching for a bar of chocolate to lift their spirits. This response is so instinctive to many of us that we don't even consider looking elsewhere for an emotional pick-me-up.

The 'Nucleus Accumbens' is the region of our brain which is responsible for the cognitive processing of pleasure and reward. This area also governs the motivation, aversion and reinforcement aspects of our behaviour and it is at the centre of all addictions.

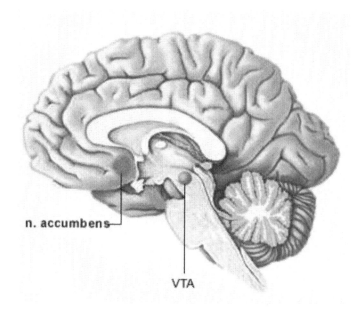

n. accumbens

VTA

Sugar produces similar effects on the Nucleus Accumbens as drugs such as nicotine, amphetamine and cocaine. As with these drugs, sugar also stimulates a higher level of dopamine production and thereby triggers the pleasure/reward process.

The higher dopamine level causes de-sensitivity in the nervous systems reaction to the stimulant, in this case sugar. This results in a higher sugar level being required to achieve the uplifting feelings a sugar boost provides. The more sugar the body needs, the stronger the cravings we experience.

The problem lies in the fact that unlike drugs, a cake, biscuit or a handful of sweets is not just socially acceptable but often, it is eaten without any negative thoughts of the damage it can cause. Aside of weight gain issues, sugar is rarely seen as an enemy of the body.

With any form of drug you are aware of the physical, neurological and emotional dangers associated with it prior to choosing to use it. None of these taboo's are considered when you pick up a bar of chocolate or glass of fruit juice, but they are just as relevant with sugar as they are with drugs.

One sweet treat here and there is not an issue; you eat your chocolate and believe that's you done for the day and you relax, quite happy in the knowledge that you have had a treat and not overindulged. Throughout the course of the day you continue with a normal eating routine.

A piece of fruit for a midday snack, an evening meal made using any number of low fat or healthy foods purchased from the supermarket, maybe a yoghurt for supper and a few cups of tea with one or two sugars, or even an artificial sweetener, nothing to worry about and all quite healthy right? Wrong.

Every one of those items listed contain sugar of some variety or another and, throughout the day they are busy satisfying the sugar cravings you may not even have realized you were having. Because we unwittingly consume so much sugar during our waking hours, it is not surprising that so many people are unknowingly addicted to sugar.

If you are still unconvinced that sugar is affecting you, try going a full day with little or no sugar intake and monitor the changes in your mood, tiredness levels, headaches and nervous shaking.

Chapter 2 – Sugar & Your Health

Once consumed, our bodies convert sugar into glucose and fructose. The glucose is then used as our main energy source. Unless you are following a low carbohydrate diet which has changed your metabolic process over to Ketosis, you will require some level of sugar in your daily diet.

According to the British National Health Service, the safe daily sugar consumption is around 5% of your daily calorie intake.

If you prefer to give up sugar completely you will need to follow a diet which is very low in carbohydrate. This will force your body into ketosis, where fat is used as an energy source rather than glucose. Before you consider this you should research Ketogenic diets thoroughly as some medical conditions are unsuitable to this form of eating. For this reason I am not recommending a complete withdrawal from sugar; that must be down to your own personal choice.

Physical Effects of Excessive Sugar Consumption

Liver Problems

Unlike glucose, the fructose which is produced from sugar is of no real benefit to us in its natural form and can only be processed by the liver. The liver converts the fructose into glycogen which it then stores for use later as and when needed. The stored glycogen is the bodies back up should its glucose levels be depleted.

This is an effective way to store energy reserves however, if we fill our bodies with too much sugar an excessive amount of fructose is directed to the liver for processing. This results in far too much glycogen being stored within the liver, overloading it and leading to a condition commonly known as 'fatty liver', (Steatosis).

Most people who have Steatosis feel no adverse symptoms and are only made aware of the condition if they have a blood test. This first stage of liver disease is relatively harmless and rarely develops further into the second stage for non alcoholics.

Normal liver

Fat liver

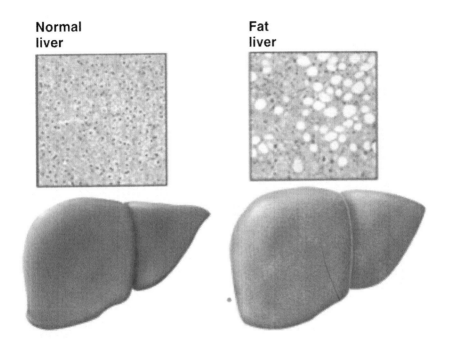

For those who are unfortunate enough for the disease to progress, the second stage is Non-Alcoholic Steatohepatitis, (NASH). This causes the liver to become inflamed because the cells within the liver are becoming damaged and dying.

NASH may or may not present symptoms of a dull ache to the right side of your stomach, just over your lower ribs. Unlike stage 1, NASH is not apparent through a blood test and largely goes unnoticed.

Stage 3 of liver disease is Fibrosis. This results in the generation of fibrous scar tissue due to the constant inflammation of the liver.

During stage 3 your liver still contains enough healthy tissue for it to function effectively and again, this stage is often not noticed, and therein hides the real danger. Stages one to three develop slowly over a period of time and as the changes are slow and gradual with symptoms being either mild or non-existent, and because the liver is still functioning well the disease often goes unnoticed.

If a sustained high sugar intake is maintained during stages 1-3, this can lead to the development of the 4th stage.

Stage four is Cirrhosis, an illness the majority of non-medically trained people associate as an illness only alcoholics develop. This is, in fact, a myth and Cirrhosis can also be caused by fatty liver.

In stage 4, the liver shrinks and becomes lumpy. This is due to the development of clumps of liver cells. The clumps are caused by the scarred tissue which has slowly developed into bands which squash together the healthy cells.

In non alcoholics, this stage takes many years to develop and it is rare for anyone below the age of 50 to suffer from it.

Insulin Resistance

Insulin Resistance is a pre-curser to the more serious Diabetes Type 2 and Metabolic Syndrome.

The hormone Insulin is essential for the body's ability to burn glucose in the blood stream. Once the body becomes resistant to the insulin's function, high levels of glucose are able to build up within the blood, which then becomes extremely toxic.

This leads to type 2 Diabetes, Obesity, Metabolic Syndrome and Heart Disease.

Cancer

Over recent years, scientists have been conducting studies into the link between cancer and glucose.

These studies have shown that high levels of blood glucose can lead to the development of various cancers and also produces the lowest rate of cancer survival in patients.

Obesity

We are all aware that excess sugar = fat. This is due to the excess glucose produced by our body is not needed to fuel our energy levels. This excess is transformed within our bodies by a process called Lipogenesis.

Lipogenesis converts the glucose into fat which it then stores for future use. If we then continue to overindulge in sugar, this becomes a constant process leading to large amounts of stored fat throughout the body.

Obesity can lead to illnesses which include:

- Heart Disease
- Osteoarthritis
- Gallbladder Problems
- High Blood Pressure
- Breathing Issues and Asthma
- Strokes
- Disturbed Sleep and/or Insomnia

Skin, Hair, Nails & Teeth

Due to the swelling caused by sugar, excessive consumption can cause the breakout of spots and boils, both on the face and the rest of the body, but this is not the only skin issue caused by sugar addiction.

Sugar actively attacks the collagen in our skin causing it to become dehydrated and dull. The lack of collagen decreases the supple and youthful look of skin and results in wrinkles and premature aging. Prolonged attacks on the collagen levels result in many deep set wrinkles which can add years to your appearance.

Excess sugar intake is also responsible for numerous rashes, yeast imbalances, skin redness and, thanks to the dehydration it causes, those hard to erase dark circles under and around the eyes.

Although it may appear unrelated to this section, poor digestion can wreak havoc with your skin. Sugar caused inflammation within the gut leading to stomach discomfort and nausea which results from an inflamed digestive system. This stops the sugar from being effectively digested and dispersed leaving it to sit and ferment within the stomach.

It is not just your skin that suffers the external effects of too much sugar. Hair and nails are made up of the protein, Keratin and both react in the same way when your body is exposed to prolonged high sugar intake. Finger and toe nails become weak with nails becoming brittle. Hair and nails suffer from breakages and quickly become noticeably unhealthy.

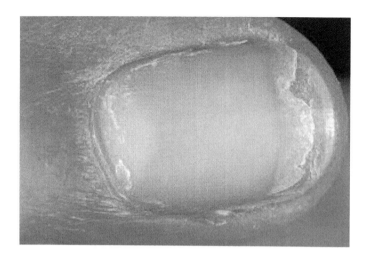

Since the turn of this century, scientists have been conducting extensive research into the links between sugar addictive and baldness. Finding have shown that insulin resistance leads to a lack of stability of the hair follicles which cause it to thin and, in some cases, fall out altogether.

Oral hygiene is an important issue for everyone but should be of particular concern to a sugar addict.
Some oral bacteria cause the sugars which coat our teeth to become almost glue-like. This 'glue' then adheres to the gums and teeth and eats away at out oral health leading to tooth decay and tooth loss.

Emotional Effects of Sugar Addiction

Emotions are extremely susceptible to the changes in blood sugar levels. Mood swings are the most commonly recognized emotional symptom of blood sugar fluctuations but anxiety, fatigue, depression and confusion are also adversely affected along with the inability to concentrate and focus.

Stress is a huge factor in the highs and lows associated with high blood sugar. Stress causes the body to release the hormones Cortisol and Epinephrine. These two hormones often cause the blood sugar level to rise and spike. If you already have a sugar addiction your levels are starting out high, add these additional spikes and the lows that follow into the equation and your emotional balance will be thrown into a tailspin.

Many people reach for a chocolate bar when they feel their energy level drop and this often results in a much needed energy boost, but it will be short lived and followed by a sugar crash. While this high and low may be felt physically for a short amount of time, the subsequent emotional disruption can last several hours.

During this time your clarity of thought will be severely diminished, your concentration will be gone and feelings of anxiety will flood your body. As these emotions begin to wane they will be replaced, or accompanied, by restlessness, hunger, irritability, anger, light-headedness, sweating and possibly slurred speech.

The easy solution is to go back to the beginning and grab another sugary snack to lift your sugar levels back up but this will simply restore the initial cycle of emotional confusion and further embed the sugar dependency into your psyche.

Chapter 3 – Cravings & Withdrawal

Mental cravings are triggered by the brains demand for dopamine production to satisfy its need for reward.

No matter what your addiction is, the cravings usually present in the form of hunger or persistent thoughts of a need for a particular type of food or drug, but as they stem from a neurological rather than physical basis, they are rarely triggered by a true need.

The cravings are produced in response to an emotional reaction such as stress, anxiety, sadness and anger and the brain reacts by triggering the need for reward. Long term emotional issues can help to fix this need for instant gratification firmly in your psyche and it becomes the instinctive go-to place in times of emotional need.

When you are also genuinely hungry, the cravings are even harder to ignore, but there are ways to counteract the need for sugar which I will go into in greater detail in the next chapter.

Withdrawal

All addictions are made up of 4 elements:

- **Binging:** Whether you have a crazy few hours of filling your body with as much sugar as possible or simply eat a large bar of chocolate or slice of cake, you are binging. Media has hyped up the concept of binging in relation to addiction and it is typically assumed to refer to long periods of consuming your drug of choice, whether that is food, alcohol or narcotics. Binging is in fact, much simpler that we have been led to believe. In its most basic definition, it means overindulging.

- **Cravings:** The need to satisfy a desire.

- **Withdrawal:** The physical and emotional effects of denying the body or mind something it feels it needs.

- **Cross-sensitization:** The most dangerous component when attempting to break an addiction. This is the replacement of one addiction with an alternative substance to ensure the cravings are satisfied.

How you choose to break a sugar addiction, or manage excess sugar consumption is a personal choice but there are two options:

Cold Turkey:
Withdrawal symptoms are more intense if sugar is cut out completely and, due to the bodies need for an energy supply, I would urge anyone considering this to research Ketogenic diets before taking this step.

Avoidance:
Avoidance relates to the removal of non natural sugars from your diet. This allows the body the ability to retain glucose as the primary energy source and reduces the effects of withdrawal. It also allows the cravings to be satiated in a small but natural way and provides the opportunity to retrain your brain as to the correct foods to request as rewards when needed.

How long the withdrawal symptoms last is dependent on individuality with factors such as how long you have been over indulging, how much sugar is consumed on a daily/weekly basis and your personality. Physical symptoms will start to ease after a week or two with some people barely noticing them at all after this time.

The psychological withdrawal is often the hardest to cope with. Your mind has spent years recognizing sugar as a reward and it typically takes around 3 weeks of consistent behavior to break a mental habit.

By replacing a high sugar fix with something that has naturally occurring sugar, you are lessening the hold in a healthier way while still managing to retrain your brain.

While many people believe that they will need to ban sweet treats from their life after breaking a sugar habit, many others have found that after the initial few months, they can introduce sweet treats back into their lives on a restrictive basis.

A small slice of cake every now and again or a couple of squares of chocolate instead of a whole chocolate bar is fine providing you have a firm grasp on the amount you consume and how often you allow yourself to eat it.

One mistake many people make when cutting down their sugar intake is to switch to artificial sugars. This will not help retrain the brain as you are still consuming something which tastes sweet. It will also prolong the withdrawal as you are denying your body the sugar it wants when it craves then feeding it to it every time you have a cup of tea.

Symptoms you may experience while withdrawing from sugar will vary in intensity from person to person and may include any or all of the following:

- Anxiety
- Irritability and Anger
- Cravings
- Low Mood
- Mood Swings
- Changes in Appetite and Taste
- Tiredness and Fatigue
- Muscular Aches
- Light Headedness
- Headaches
- Shaking
- Sleep Disruption or Insomnia
- Feeling of Fake Hunger

Chapter 4 – Changing your Habits

Before you begin to change your eating habits you need to decide if you are going to use the cold turkey or avoidance method. Once you have established this, I found a great way to reinforce the decision is to wait a day or two before starting.

In this first day or two, eat as you normally would and keep a diary of everything you eat. At the end of the first day, look through your food list and sum up how many grams of sugar you have consumed that day. Then take a normal bag of granulated sugar and weigh out that amount.

Trust me; it is a shock to the system when you can physically see how much sugar you have poured into yourself in one day.

What is sugar?
When we think of sugar, the picture that comes to mind is normal household sugar that we use in our cup of tea. But that is only one type of sugar.

Sugar is a short-chain carbohydrate that has a sweet taste, although many of these carbohydrates don't really taste sweet.

Naturally occurring sugars are found in many fruits and vegetables and milk. These are the natural sugars and it is these foods that should provide you with your daily sugar intake.

The 4 main sugars are:

- **Sucrose:** This is the sugar that is used daily to sweeten drinks, breakfast cereals, in baking and all other manner of foods. It is made from a combination of glucose and fructose. While this is naturally found in some fruits and vegetables, the manufactured sucrose comes from sugar cane or sugar beet but by the time it reaches our homes it is no longer in a natural form.

- **Fructose:** Along with glucose, this is naturally occurring in fruits and vegetables and is also the cause of the sweet taste of natural honey.

- **Lactose:** Lactose is naturally occurring and is derived from milk. A natural dairy product with no added sugars will taste less sweet than the more manufactured varieties but will still contain lactose.

- **Maltose:** Maltose is derived from Malt and is found in many beers and malt based drinks.

These 4 sugars are the easiest to recognize in the ingredients list of a food product, but many others are hidden behind fancy names. As a general rule, anything that ends in 'OSE' is a sugar.

Other hidden sugars include:
- Cane
- Dextrin & Malt dextrin
- Dextrin
- Demarara Sugar
- Barley Malt
- Syrups
- Fruit Concentrate or Juice
- Ethyl Maltol
- Maple
- Turbinado

Plan Your Diet
Being conscious of what you are eating and when will help in the first few weeks. If you are aware of what you will be eating for your lunch, main meal and breakfast on a daily basis you will alleviate the confusion caused from changing your eating habits.

Preparing your menu up front will help you to avoid turning to your usual food choices and if you ensure there are plenty of sugar free snacks around, or foods that contain natural sugars, you will be able to satisfy your cravings in a gentle way while keeping hunger at bay.

Do not be tricked into buying low fat foods. To ensure taste, these foods are packed with hidden sugars.

Stop or cut down on the sugar in your hot beverages. This may taste a little unpleasant at first but taste-buds adapt and within a week or two you won't miss the sugary taste.

Foods which are labeled as 'sugar free' often contain artificial sweeteners.

Eat plenty of proteins to keep you feeling full for longer.

When cooking, use herbs and spices in place of sugars to add flavor.

Eat oats and whole wheat products instead of white bread, white pasta and white rice.

Beating the Cravings

Be kind to yourself. Every now and again give yourself a treat. Choose to have 1 biscuit, a small piece of chocolate or a bite sized bun instead of a large cupcake. Denying yourself all the little pleasures will only make you crave them more. The trick is how you think about the treats.

If you pick up a tiny piece of chocolate it is unlikely your brain will accept that as a reward. Instead, place your treat on a small plate along with a handful of nuts, some slices of carrot and a few raisins and make yourself a small picnic.

Exercise: You don't need to go mad with exercise but a small burst of physical activity will release endorphins that allow you to feel good. This takes the focus of reward away and you are left feeling great. Choose fruit as a snack.

Hunger is stressful on the body and as stress triggers cravings, you need to eat small and often. Instead of 3 big meals, try eating 5 smaller meals throughout the day.

Chapter 5 – High Sugar Foods

The best way to ensure you are not eating any hidden sugars is to use natural ingredients to make your own meals. Below is a list of food and drinks that are high in sugar and should be avoided.

- Soft drinks
- Fizzy Drinks
- Sweets
- Jams
- Syrup and Treacle
- Sugar and Artificially Modified Honey
- Cakes
- Biscuits
- Pastries
- Ice-cream
- Alcohol
- Confectionary
- Pre-prepared Sauces
- Canned Goods
- Convenience Foods

Try to use only foods that are naturally low in sugar when cooking or planning your menu.

Meat, eggs, beans, seeds and nuts are all good sources of vitamins and minerals and will go a long way to keeping you away the hunger pangs. Low sugar vegetables include Olives, spinach, beetroot, green vegetables, turnips, asparagus, lettuce and other salad vegetables.

If you make your own sauces or casserole mixes etc, you can avoid all the hidden, added sugars which are found in convenience foods. While this will extend the initial preparation and cooking times, if you make large batches and freeze them into individual portions, you will have healthy, ready-made sauces on hand whenever you need them, and they will taste great too.

Chapter 6 – Low Sugar Recipes

Banana Pancakes

Serves 2

Ingredients:

2 ripe bananas

2 Eggs

1 cup chopped fresh fruit

¼ cup almond milk

½ cup flour (whole wheat)

¼ tsp salt

½ tsp baking powder

Preparation:

- Mash the bananas
- Whisk Eggs and stir in flour, salt, baking powder and almond milk
- Whisk in the mashed bananas until you reach a smooth, pouring consistency
- Lightly oil a frying pan and heat over a medium heat
- Pour in roughly 4 tablespoons of the batter mixture and cook for a few minutes until brown underneath
- Turn over the pancake and cook till browned
- Serve with a sprinkle of chopped fruit

Buttermilk Pancakes with Blueberries

Serves 6
Ingredients:
   1½ cup whole wheat flour
1½ tsp baking powder
½ tsp baking soda
¼ tsp salt
1½ cups unsweetened buttermilk
¼ cup freshly squeezed grapefruit juice
2 eggs
1 cup blueberries
Preparation:
- Add baking powder, flour, baking soda and salt to a bowl and mix together
- Whisk eggs and add grapefruit juice and buttermilk. Whisk together
- Add flour mix to the egg mix and whisk to a smooth consistency
- Lightly oil a frying pan and heat over a medium heat
- Add ¼ cup of batter to the frying pan and cook until the batter begins to bubble and lift from the pan
- Sprinkle with blueberries and cook until brown on the underside
- Flip over pancakes and continue to cook until browned

Sweet and Sour Chicken

Serves 4
Ingredients:

1 lb chicken breast meat (chopped)
¾ cup sesame seeds
2 cups fresh pineapple chunks
1 small onion
3 stalks celery

Sauce Ingredients:

½ cup unsweetened apricot jam
3 tbsp freshly squeezed lime juice
2 tbsp shredded coconut

Preparation:

- Preheat oven to 375°f
- Coat chopped chicken with sesame seeds and place on an ovenproof tray
- Cook in oven for 20 minutes
- Chop onion and celery and lightly fry over a medium heat for 5 – 10 minutes
- Mix together apricot jam, shredded coconut and lime juice

- Just before the vegetables have finished cooking, stir in half of the sauce. Remove vegetables from the pan and set aside.
- Return the pan to the heat and add the remaining sauce
- Stir chicken into the pan and cook for a further 2 minutes
- Add the vegetables back to the pan and stir well

Serve with brown rice

BBQ Pulled Chicken

Serves 4 – 6
Ingredients:
2 lb 9oz chicken breast
6 peaches, peeled, de-stoned and chopped
2 garlic cloves, peeled and chopped
$1/3$ cup unsweetened tomato paste
½ cup chicken stock
1 tbsp mustard
1 tbsp apple cider vinegar
½ tbsp olive oil
1 tbsp paprika
¼ tsp ground cumin
½ tsp salt

Preparation:

- Puree chopped peaches
- Mix together all ingredients except chicken
- Add mixed ingredients to a pan and bring to the boil, reduce heat and simmer for 1 hour
- Allow to cool slightly then add sauce to a blender and blend until smooth
- While the sauce is simmering, add chicken breasts to a pan and cover with water
- Bring to the boil and reduce to a simmer for 30 – 40 minutes
- Drain water and place chicken on a chopping board
- Shred the chicken and add to the sauce and stir well
- Serve with brown rice or on a large burger bun with salad

Pork Casserole

Serves 6

Ingredients:

500g dried haricot beans
7 cloves chopped garlic
5 sprigs fresh thyme (chopped)
3 sprigs fresh rosemary (chopped)
1 bay leaf
1 tbsp rapeseed oil
1 medium onion, (chopped)
1 large carrot (chopped)
2 tsp butter
700g pork (diced)
125ml white wine
230g unsweetened canned chopped tomatoes

Preparation:

- Haricot beans will need to be covered with water and soaked overnight
- Drain beans and add to a pan and cover with 2 litres water
- Add 3 cloves garlic, 2 sprigs chopped thyme and 1 sprig chopped rosemary and bring to the boil
- Reduce to a simmer for 1½ hours (top up water as needed)
- In a large ovenproof pot, heat oil and add onions and carrots

- Fry over a medium heat for 5 minutes then add butter and stir in the remaining garlic and fry for 2 minutes
- Add pork and cook until browned
- Pour wine into the pot and allow to cook for a further 2 minutes
- Stir in the remaining thyme and rosemary, bay leaf and tomatoes and season with salt and pepper. Continue cooking for 3 minutes then remove from heat.
- Preheat oven to 180°c
- Drain the beans but retain the liquid
- Sieve liquid and stir beans back into it then add to ovenproof pot and stir well. Bring back to the boil and cook for a further 30 minutes
- Remove pot from stove and place into the preheated oven for 1½ hours
- Optional: 15 minutes before removing from oven, sprinkle with breadcrumbs for a tasty crust

Spicy Meatballs

Serves 4
Ingredients:
1 onion, halved and sliced
2 chopped garlic cloves
1 large bell pepper, quartered, deseeded & chopped
1 tsp ground cumin
2-3 tsp chilli paste
300ml no added sugar chicken stock
400g can no added sugar cherry tomatoes
400g can no added sugar red kidney beans, drained
1 avocado, de-stoned, peeled and chopped
Juice of ½ a lime
Meatball Ingredients:
500g turkey or beef mince
50g porridge oats
2 spring onions, finely chopped
1 tsp ground cumin
1 tsp coriander
1 tsp oil

Preparation:

- Add mince, spring onions, oats, cumin and coriander to a mixing bowl and stir together.
- Shape into 12 balls
- Heat oil in a frying pan and add meatballs, turning frequently, and cook until browned
- Remove meatballs from the pan and set aside
- Return the pan to the heat and add bell pepper, onion and garlic and cook for 2 – 3 minutes until softened.
- Stir in chilli paste and cumin then add chicken stock and bring to just below boiling
- Add meatballs back into the pan and simmer on a low heat for 10 – 12 minutes
- Add tomatoes and beans to the pan and stir. Cook for a further 2 – 3 minutes
- In a separate bowl, stir lime juice over the avocado
- Serves meatballs with pasta and garnish with avocado and lime

Fish Stew

Serves 6 – 8

Ingredients:
3 tbsp olive or vegetable oil
1 large onion (chopped)
2 cloves garlic (finely chopped)
1 red chilli (finely chopped)
2 tbsp no added sugar tomato paste
1 kg chopped tomatoes
200ml white cooking wine
350ml no added sugar fish stock
Zest of 1 orange
1 kg skinless cod or halibut
400g raw prawns (de-veined and peeled)
500g clams
¼ cup chopped fresh parsley

Preparation:

- Heat the oil in a large, deep frying pan over a medium heat
- Add onion and fry for 4 – 5 minutes until softened
- Stir in chilli and garlic and cook for a further 2 minutes
- Stir in tomatoes and tomato puree and increase the heat, stirring continuously for 10 – 15 minutes
- Pour in the wine and stir well. Continue to cooks for a further 10 minutes
- Add fish stock and orange zest and stir well
- Reduce heat to a low simmer and add cod then cook for an additional 5 minutes
- Stir in clams and prawns and continue cooking for around 5 minutes until the clams have opened
- Garnish with parsley and serve

Onion Soup

Serves 4
Ingredients:
1 tbsp olive oil
500g sliced or chopped onions
1 sliced leek
4 cups no added sugar beef stock
2 cloves garlic (chopped)
Pinch of chopped fresh thyme
1 tbsp rice wine vinegar
1 cup red wine
Pinch salt and pepper

Preparation:
- Heat oil over a medium to high heat and add onions and leek
- Reduce heat and fry gently for 20 minutes, stirring 2 – 3 times
- Add garlic and rice vinegar and stir well. Continue cooking for a further minute
- Stir in red wine and thyme and cook for a further 2 – 3 minutes
- Season with salt & pepper
- Simmer for 20 – 30 minutes

Chicken Noodle Soup

Serves 2

Ingredients:

2 cups no added sugar chicken stock

1 cooked chicken breast, (shredded)

2 tbsp no added sugar soy sauce

2 cloves chopped garlic

2 tsp chopped fresh ginger

2 chopped spring onions

1 egg

200g fine noodles

2 tsp sesame oil

1 red chilli (chopped)

Preparation:

- Add chicken stock to a large pan and stir in ginger, chilli and garlic
- Bring to the boil
- Stir in soy sauce and sesame oil
- Add noodles and reduce heat to a simmer and cook for 5 minutes
- Stir in shredded chicken and spring onions
- Whisk egg in a separate bowl
- Remove pan from heat and quickly stir in the beaten egg. Stir continuously for 30 seconds to ensure egg cooks evenly through the soup
- Add to bowls and serve

Tuna Pasta

Serves 4

Ingredients:
1 tsp olive oil
2 bell peppers, sliced and de-seeded
2 cloves chopped garlic
½ tsp crushed chilli
800g canned no added sugar chopped tomatoes
50g pitted olives (chopped)
250g wholemeal pasta
400g canned tuna in spring water (drained)
2 tbsp grated parmesan cheese
25g wholemeal breadcrumbs

Preparation:
- In a large saucepan, heat olive oil over a medium to high heat
- Add peppers and cook for 5 minutes
- Stir in garlic and chillies and cook for a further 30 seconds
- Add canned tomatoes, a p inch of salt and pepper and olives and stir well
- Bring to the boil then reduce heat and simmer for 10 minutes
- In a separate pan, add pasta and cover with water

- Bring to the boil then reduce heat and simmer until cooked
- Preheat the grill
- Drain pasta and add to the sauce. Stir in well
- Stir in Tuna and cook for 2 minutes then remove from heat
- Empty the saucepan into an ovenproof dish and sprinkle with breadcrumbs and parmesan cheese
- Place under the grill and grill for 3 – 5 minutes until breadcrumbs are golden and cheese has melted
- Serve with salad

Lamb & Pumpkin Soup

Serves 6
Ingredients:
450g lamb, diced
1 large onion, diced
2 tbsp olive oil
1 large carrot, chopped
3 cloves garlic, crushed
½ tsp chilli powder
2 cups pumpkin, chopped
1 can no added sugar cannellini beans, drained and rinsed
1 tsp lemon zest
1 tsp finely chopped fresh ginger
4 cups no added sugar beef stock
2 cups water
2 tbsp chopped fresh coriander
Pinch salt & Pepper

Spices:
½ tsp cumin
Pinch cinnamon
½ tsp turmeric
½ tsp ground cloves

Preparation:

- Mix together cumin, cinnamon, turmeric and ground cloves and set to one side
- Heat a little olive oil in a medium saucepan over a medium heat
- Add onions and cook for 8 – 10 minutes
- In a small to medium frying pan, heat a little more olive oil and add lamb
- Cook on a medium heat, stirring occasionally, until browned.
- Remove from heat and add lamb to the saucepan with onions
- Sprinkle lamb and onions with the mixed spices and cook for 30 seconds, stirring continuously
- Stir stock and water into the lamb and onions
- Add ginger, garlic and chilli and stir well
- Allow to heat to a medium to fast simmer
- Add carrots, pumpkin, beans, lemon zest and salt and pepper
- Leave to simmer for 1½ hours, (top up with water if required)

Almond & Berry Cupcakes

Makes around 16 – 18 muffins

Ingredients:

1 cup rice flour

1 cup corn meal or almond meal

1 tbsp baking powder

¼ tsp salt

1 ripe banana

¼ cup vegetable oil

3 large eggs

1 cup milk

1 tsp vanilla essence

1 cup blackberries (or any berry of your choice)

¾ cup chopped almonds

Preparation:

- Preheat oven to 400 °f
- Place cupcake cases in a bun tray
- Mix together flour, corn meal, baking powder and salt
- In a separate bowl mash banana and whisk together with eggs
- Add oil, milk and vanilla essence to the egg mix and whisk together
- Gradually add the flour mix to the egg mix, whisking slowly until it forms a smooth mixture
- Stir in berries and spoon into cupcake cases

- Sprinkle with chopped almonds and place in the oven for 15 – 20 minutes
- Allow to cool before eating

Banana Bread

Ingredients:

2 large eggs

2 large bananas (mashed)

1/2 cup unsweetened apple sauce

1/4 cup milk

1 tsp vanilla extract

1 cup white flour

1 cup whole wheat flour

1 tsp baking soda

1 tsp baking powder

1 tsp salt

1/2 tsp cinnamon

1/2 tsp nutmeg

Preparation:

- Preheat oven to 350°c
- Whisk the eggs until fluffy.
- Mix together the apple sauce and mashed bananas and add to the egg
- Add milk and vanilla extract and stir well
- In a separate bowl mix together white flour, whole wheat flour, baking soda, baking powder, cinnamon, nutmeg and salt
- Stir into the egg mixture and mix well

- Pour into a greased or lined loaf tin and bake for 45 minutes
- Allow to cool before slicing

Fruit & Coconut Ice Cream

Serves
Ingredients:
2 cans unsweetened coconut milk
4 cups chopped melon
¼ cup fresh lime juice
2 cups fresh or frozen berries

Preparation:
- Add melon, lime juice and berries to a blend and puree together
- Line a small, deep baking tray with greaseproof paper
- Pour coconut milk into line baking tray and place in the freezer for 1 – 2 hours
- Remove frozen coconut milk from freezer and break into pieces
- Add coconut milk pieces to the blender and blend for a few seconds at a time until it starts to form into a creamy mixture
- Add fruit puree and blend for 30 seconds
- Empty ice cream into a greaseproof lined tub and return to the freezer for at least 1 hour

Conclusion

Thank you again for downloading this book!

I hope this book was able to help you to understand the dangers and adverse effects of consuming high levels of sugar on a regular basis and help lead in the right direction when considering meals, snacks and drinks.

The next step upon successful completion of this book is to try out some of the low sugar recipes and begin your journey to a healthier mind and body with delicious meals and snacks.

Finally, if you enjoyed this book, please click the link below to share your thoughts and post a review on Amazon. It'd be greatly appreciated!

Thank you and good luck!

Printed in Great Britain
by Amazon